"There are gems of thought that
are ageless and eternal."
Cicero
Born 106 B.C.—Arpino, Italy

Copyright 2021 by Cathy Byrd

Published in the United States by: 108 Stitches Entertainment LLC

Proceeds to benefit Open Arms Foundation 501c3

life-is-a-miracle.com

All rights reserved. No part of this book may be reproduced by any mechanical, photographic, or electronic process, without prior written permission of the publisher.

1st edition, January 2022

Tradepaper ISBN: 978-0-578-33946-7

E-book ISBN: 978-0-578-33949-8

LIFE IS
A MIRACLE

LIFE IS A MIRACLE

a collection of words to live by

CATHY BYRD

Open Arms Foundation 501c3 life-is-a-miracle.com

for Charlotte and Christian

CONTENTS

INTRODUCTION	**xiii**
I ADVENTURE	**1**
II ATHLETICS	**4**
III BEAUTY	**7**
IV CHARACTER	**9**
V CHILDHOOD	**11**
VI COMMUNITY	**14**
VII CONFIDENCE	**17**
VIII COURAGE	**19**
IX CURIOSITY	**22**
X DEATH	**24**
XI FAITH	**27**
XII FORGIVENESS	**29**

CONTENTS

XIII	FRIENDSHIP	31
XIV	GOD	33
XV	GRATITUDE	35
XVI	HAPPINESS	37
XVII	HOME/FAMILY	39
XVIII	HOPE	41
XIX	HUMBLENESS	43
XX	INTUITION	45
XXI	JOY	47
XXII	KINDNESS	49
XXIII	LETTING GO	51
XXIV	LIFE PURPOSE	53
XXV	LOVE	56
XXVI	MANIFESTATION	58
XXVII	THE MIND	60

CONTENTS

XXVIII	MYSTERY OF LIFE	63
XXIX	NATURE	65
XXX	PEACE	68
XXXI	PERSEVERANCE	70
XXXII	POSSIBILITY	73
XXXIII	PRAYERS	75
XXXIV	SLEEP/DREAMS	79
XXXV	SOLITUDE	81
XXXVI	SUCCESS	83
XXXVII	SYNCHRONICITY/MAGIC	86
XXXVIII	EXTRAS	89

INTRODUCTION

Life is a miracle. Of this we can be sure.

Each of us come into the world through the miracle of life—unconcerned and unaware of the universal struggles and questions that have perplexed mankind since the beginning of time.

Before too long, we are faced with such questions ourselves. What do we aspire to? What do we believe in? What do we want to do before we die?

It is my hope that this collection of the greatest thoughts, ideas, and philosophies that have come down to us through the ages will touch, move, and inspire us all to find meaning and purpose in our own lives.

May these kernels of wisdom, these universal truths that withstand the test of time, be the breadcrumbs that help us find our way home to who we truly are and what we are capable of becoming and doing at our very best.

Cathy Byrd

ADVENTURE

"The chances you take, the people you meet, the
people you love, the faith that you have.
That's what's going to define you."
Denzel Washington
Born 1954—Mount Vernon, New York

"I can choose to be a victim of the world or an
adventurer in search of a treasure. It's all a
question of how I live my life."
Paulo Coelho
Born 1947—Rio de Janeiro, Brazil

"The greatest adventure is living
the life of your dreams."
Oprah Winfrey
Born 1954—Kosciusko, Mississippi

"Do not go where the path may lead, go instead
where there is no path and leave a trail."
Ralph Waldo Emerson
Born 1803—Boston, Massachusetts

"Be not the slave of your own past—plunge into the sublime seas, dive deep, and swim far, so you shall come back with new self-respect, with new power, and with an advanced experience that shall explain and overlook the old."
Ralph Waldo Emerson
Born 1803—Boston, Massachusetts

"The purpose of life is to live it, to taste experience to the utmost, to reach out eagerly and without fear for newer and richer experience."
Eleanor Roosevelt
Born 1884—New York, New York

"Life is either a daring adventure or nothing. To keep our faces toward change and behave like free spirits in the presence of fate is strength undefeatable."
Helen Keller
Born 1880—Tuscumbia, Alabama

"Twenty years from now you will be more disappointed by the things that you didn't do than by the ones you did. So, throw off the bowlines, sail away from safe harbor, catch the trade winds in your sails. Explore, Dream, Discover."
Mark Twain
Born 1835—Florida, Missouri

"We didn't realize we were making memories.
We just knew we were having fun."
Winnie the Pooh
A.A. Milne
Born 1882—London, United Kingdom

"Read. The book is still the greatest
manmade machine of all—not the car,
not the TV, not the smartphone. "
Ken Burns
Born 1953—Brooklyn, New York

"A bird in a cage is safe but God
didn't create birds for that."
Paulo Coelho
Born 1947—Rio de Janeiro, Brazil

"We shall not cease from exploration
And the end of all our exploring
Will be to arrive where we started
And know the place for the first time."
T.S. Eliot
Born 1888—St. Louis, Missouri

ATHLETICS

"Everything I know most surely about morality and duty, I owe to football (soccer)."
Albert Camus
Born 1913—French Algeria

"Don't let the fear of striking out keep you from playing the game."
Babe Ruth
Born 1895—Baltimore, Maryland

"I have self-doubt. I have insecurity. I have fear of failure. We all have self-doubt. You don't deny it, but you also don't capitulate to it. You embrace it."
Kobe Bryant
Born 1978—Philadelphia, Pennsylvania

"Progress always involves risks. You can't steal second base and keep your foot on first."
Robert Quillen
Born 1887—Syracuse, Kansas

LIFE IS A MIRACLE

"I see great things in baseball. It's our game–
the American game. It will take our people
out-of-doors, fill them with oxygen, give them
a larger physical stoicism. Tend to relieve us
from being a nervous, dyspeptic set. Repair
these losses, and be a blessing to us."
Walt Whitman
Born 1819—West Hills, New York

"I love that kids are building confidence
on and off the court and unlocking
their potential through sport."
Kobe Bryant
Born 1978—Philadelphia, Pennsylvania

"I had three rules for my players:
No profanity.
Don't criticize a teammate.
Never be late."
John Wooden
Born 1910—Hall, Indiana

"There may be people that have more talent
than you, but there's no excuse for anyone
to work harder than you do."
Derek Jeter
Born 1974—Pequannock, New Jersey

> "The measure of who we are is
> what we do with what we have."
> **Vince Lombardi**
> *Born 1913—Brooklyn, New York*

> "Great things come from hard work
> and perseverance. No excuses."
> **Kobe Bryant**
> *Born 1978—Philadelphia, Pennsylvania*

> "Make sure your worst enemy doesn't
> live between your own two ears."
> **Laird Hamilton**
> *Born 1964—San Francisco, California*

> "Winning isn't everything—but wanting to win is."
> **Vince Lombardi**
> *Born 1913—Brooklyn, New York*

> "Surround yourself with people who
> will leap out of the dugout should
> you ever charge the mound."
> **BASEBALLISM**

BEAUTY

"Beauty is not in the face, beauty is a light in the heart."
Khalil Gibran
Born 1883—Bsharri, Lebanon

"Life is not measured by the number of breaths we take, but by the moments that take our breath away."
Maya Angelou
Born 1928—St. Louis, Missouri

"Everything has beauty, but not everyone sees it."
Confucius
Born 551 BC—Jining, China

"For beautiful eyes, look for the good in others."
Audrey Hepburn
Born 1929—Ixelles, Belgium

"Don't wait for someone to bring you flowers, plant your own garden and decorate your own soul."
Luther Burbank
Born 1849—Lancaster, Massachusetts

"A person who has good thoughts cannot ever by ugly. You can have a wonky nose and a crooked mouth and a double chin and stick-out teeth, but if you have good thoughts they will shine out of your face like sunbeams and you will always look lovely."
Roald Dahl
Born 1916—Cardiff, UK

"The best and most beautiful things in the world cannot be seen or even touched. They must be felt with the heart."
Helen Keller
Born 1880—Tuscumbia, Alabama

"The whole world is an art gallery when you're mindful. There are beautiful things everywhere--and they're free."
Charles Tart
Born 1937—Morrisville, Pennsylvania

IV

CHARACTER

"You can easily judge the character of a man by how he treats those who can do nothing for him."
Johann Wolfgang von Goethe
Born 1749—Frankfurt, Germany

"It is in the character of very few men to honor without envy a friend who has prospered."
Aeschylus
Born 525—Eleusis, Greece

"Be more concerned with your character than your reputation, because your character is what you really are, while your reputation is merely what others think you are."
John Wooden
Born 1910—Hall, Indiana

"Great minds discuss ideas; average minds discuss events; small minds discuss people."
Eleanor Roosevelt
Born 1884—New York, New York

> "There is no room in baseball for discrimination.
> It is our national pastime and a game for all."
> **Lou Gehrig**
> *Born 1903—New York, New York*

> "Be independent of the good opinion of other people."
> **Abraham Maslow**
> *Born 1908—Brooklyn, New York*

> "But the fruit of the spirit is love, joy, peace, patience, kindness, goodness, faithfulness, gentleness, self-control; against such things there is no law."
> **5 Galatians 22-23**

> "Is it the TRUTH?
> Is it FAIR to all concerned?
> Will it build GOODWILL
> and BETTER FRIENDSHIPS?
> Will it be BENEFICIAL to all concerned?"
> **Rotary International Four-Way Test**
> **of the things we think, say or do**

CHILDHOOD

"Grown men may learn from very little children,
for the hearts of little children are pure, and,
therefore, the Great Spirit may show to them
many things which older people miss."
Black Elk
Born 1863—Powder River, Montana

"Every child comes with the message that
God is not yet discouraged of man."
Rabindranath Tagore
Born 1861—Kolkata India

"See that you don't look down on one of these little
ones, because I tell you that in heaven their angels
continually view the face of my Father in heaven."
Matthew 18:10

"Every child is an artist. The problem is how
to remain an artist once we grow up."
Pablo Picasso
Born 1881—Malaga, Spain

> "I wept because I was re-experiencing the enthusiasm of my childhood; I was once again a child, and nothing in the world could cause me harm."
> **Paulo Coelho**
> *Born 1947—Rio de Janeiro, Brazil*

> "It is not what you do for your children, but what you have taught them to do for themselves, that will make them good human beings."
> **Ann Landers**
> *Born 1918—Sioux City, Iowa*

> "Each second we live is a new and unique moment of the universe, a moment that never was before and will never be again. And what do we teach our children? We teach them that two and two makes four, and that Paris is the capital of France. When will we also teach them what they are? We should say to each of them: Do you know what you are? You are a marvel. You are unique. In all the world there is no other child exactly like you. You may become a Shakespeare, a Michelangelo, a Beethoven. You have the capacity for anything. Yes, you are a marvel. And when you grow up, can you then harm another who is, like you, a marvel? You must cherish one another. You must work—we all must work—to make this world worthy of its children."
> **Pablo Casals**
> *Born 1876—Vendrell, Spain*

On Children

"Your children are not your children.
They are the sons and daughters of
Life's longing for itself.
They come through you but not from you,
And though they are with you yet they belong not to you.
You may give them your love but not your thoughts,
For the have their own thoughts.
You may house their bodies but not their souls,
For their souls dwell in the house of tomorrow,
Which you cannot visit, not even in your dreams."

Kahlil Gibran
Born 1883—Bsharri, Lebanon

VI

COMMUNITY

"Alone we can do so little;
together we can do so much."
Helen Keller
Born 1880—Tuscumbia, Alabama

"A life is not important except in
the impact it has on other lives."
Jackie Robinson
Born 1919—Cairo, Georgia

"The fact is that people are good.
Give people affection and security, and
they will give affection and be secure
in their feelings and their behavior."
Abraham Maslow
Born 1908—Brooklyn, New York

"When 'i' is replaced with 'we'
even illness becomes wellness."
Malcolm X
Born 1925—Omaha, Nebraska

LIFE IS A MIRACLE

"I've learned that people will forget what you said, people will forget what you did, but people will never forget how you made them feel."
Maya Angelou
Born 1928—St. Louis, Missouri

"Never underestimate the ability of a group of thoughtful and dedicated people to change the world."
Cathy Byrd
Born 1967—Pine Bluff, Arkansas

"When I was a boy and I would see scary things in the news, my mother would say to me, 'Look for the helpers. You will always find people who are helping.'"
Fred Rogers
Born 1928—Latrobe, Pennsylvania

"Unless someone like YOU cares a whole awful lot, nothing is going to get better. It's not."
Dr. Seuss
Born 1904—Springfield, Massachusetts

"Connect with people who remind you of what you truly are."
Ralph Smart
Born 1986—London, United Kingdom

> "You may say I'm a dreamer, but I'm not
> the only one. I hope someday you'll join us.
> And the world will live as one."
> **John Lennon**
> *Born 1940—Liverpool, United Kingdom*

> "As human beings, our job in life is to help people
> realize how rare and valuable each one of us
> really is, that each of us has something that
> no one else has—or ever will have—
> something inside that is unique to all time."
> **Fred Rogers**
> *Born 1928—Latrobe, Pennsylvania*

> "Compassion, goodwill, common sense,
> understanding, and love are just a few
> of the things in life that are free."
> Use them.
> **Wilt Chamberlain**
> *Born 1936—Philadelphia, Pennsylvania*

> "It's not always easy and sometimes life
> can be deceiving. I'll tell you one thing,
> it's always better when we're together."
> **Jack Johnson**
> *Born 1975—North Shore, Hawaii*

VII

CONFIDENCE

"It is confidence in our bodies, minds, and spirits that allows us to keep looking for new adventures."
Oprah Winfrey
Born 1954—Kosciusko, Mississippi

"You are braver than you believe,
stronger than you seem,
and smarter than you think."
A.A. Milne
Born 1882—London, United Kingdom

"You just need one person to believe
in you (if that person is you)."
Kenneth Cole
Born 1954—Brooklyn, New York

"Just believe in yourself. Even if you don't, pretend
that you do and, at some point, you will."
Venus Williams
Born 1980—Lynnwood, California

> "As soon as you trust yourself,
> you will know how to live."
> **Johann Wolfgang von Goethe**
> *Born 1749—Frankfurt, Germany*

> "Go confidently in the direction of your dreams.
> Live the life you have imagined."
> **Henry David Thoreau**
> *Born 1817—Concord, Massachusetts*

> "If you are insecure, guess what?
> The rest of the world is too.
> Do not overestimate the competition
> and underestimate yourself.
> You are better than you think."
> **Harv Eker**
> *Born 1954—Toronto, Canada*

> "It's your road, and yours alone. Others may walk
> it with you, but no one can walk it for you."
> **Rumi**
> *Born 1207—Balkh, Afghanistan*

> "The whole problem with the world is that fools
> and fanatics are always so certain of themselves,
> and wiser people so full of doubts."
> **Bertrand Russell**
> *Born 1872—Trelleck, United Kingdom*

VIII

COURAGE

"If you are afraid to fail, you will never do the things you are capable of doing."
John Wooden
Born 1910—Hall, Indiana

"Life shrinks or expands in proportion to one's courage."
Anais Nin
Born 1903—Neuilly-sur-Seine, France

"Out of suffering have emerged the strongest souls; the most massive characters are seared with scars."
Kahlil Gibran
Born 1883—Bsharri, Lebanon

"Security is mostly a superstition. It does not exist in nature, nor do the children of men as a whole experience it. Life is either a daring adventure, or nothing."
Helen Keller
Born 1880—Tuscumbia, Alabama

"Everything you want is on the other side of fear."
Jack Canfield
Born 1944—Fort Worth, Texas

"Each time we face our fear, we gain strength, courage, and confidence in the doing."
Theodore Roosevelt
Born 1858—Manhattan, New York

"Courage is resistance to fear, mastery of fear, not absence of fear."
Mark Twain
Born 1835—Florida, Missouri

"Hang in there. Today is the tomorrow you were so worried about yesterday. Don't give up, just keep in there, just keep fighting. Be bold and mighty forces will come to your aid."
Anthony Hopkins
Born 1937—Margam, United Kingdom

"Though my soul may set in darkness, it will rise in perfect light; I have loved the stars too fondly to be fearful of the night."
Sarah Williams
Born 1837—London, United Kingdom

THE MAN IN THE ARENA

"It is not the critic who counts; not the man who points out how the strong man stumbles, or where the doer of deeds could have done them better. The credit belongs to the man who is actually in the arena, whose face is marred by dust and sweat and blood; who strives valiantly; who errs, who comes short again and again, because there is no effort without error and shortcoming; but who does actually strive to do the deeds; who knows great enthusiasms, the great devotions; who spends himself in a worthy cause; who at the best knows in the end the triumph of high achievement, and who at the worst, if he fails, at least fails while daring greatly, so that his place shall never be with those cold and timid souls who neither know victory nor defeat."

Theodore Roosevelt
Born 1858—Manhattan, New York

IX

CURIOSITY

"The important thing is not to stop questioning. Curiosity has its own reason for existing."
Albert Einstein
Born 1879—Ulm, Germany

"Life was meant to be lived, and curiosity must be kept alive. One must never, for whatever reason, turn his back on life."
Eleanor Roosevelt
Born 1884—New York, New York

"Sell your cleverness and purchase bewilderment."
Rumi
Born 1207—Balkh, Afghanistan

"Be a loner. That gives you time to wonder, to search for the truth. Have holy curiosity. Make your life worth living."
Albert Einstein
Born 1879—Ulm, Germany

LIFE IS A MIRACLE

"I think at a child's birth, if a mother could ask a fairy godmother to endow it with the most useful gift, that would be curiosity."
Eleanor Roosevelt
Born 1884—New York, New York

"It ain't what you don't know that gets you into trouble. It's what you know for sure that just ain't so."
Mark Twain
Born 1835—Florida, Missouri

"In the word question, there is a beautiful word—quest. I love that word."
Elie Wiesel
Born 1928—Sighetu Marmației, Romania

"Follow your bliss and don't be afraid, and doors will open where you didn't know they were going to be."
Joseph Campbell
Born 1904—White Plains, New York

"Live your questions now, and perhaps even without knowing it, you will live along some distant day into your answers."
Rainer Maria Rilke
Born 1975—Prague, Czech Republic

DEATH

"It is not death that a man should fear, but he should fear never beginning to live."
Marcus Aurelius
Born 121—Rome, Italy

"I'd like to get away from earth awhile. And then come back to it and begin again."
Robert Frost
Born 1874—San Francisco, California

"Dust thou art, to dust returnest
Was not spoken of the soul."
Henry Wadsworth Longfellow
Born 1807—Portland, Maine

"Don't be dismayed at good-byes. A farewell is necessary before you can meet again. And meeting gain, after moments or lifetimes, is certain for those who are friends."
Richard Bach
Born 1936—Oak Park, Illinois

"It's so silly," [Teddy] said. "All you do is get the heck out of your body when you die. My gosh, everybody's done it thousands and thousands of times. Just because they don't remember it doesn't mean they haven't done it. It's silly."
J.D. Salinger
Born 1919—Manhattan, NY

"I did not begin when I was born, nor when I was conceived. I have been growing, developing, through incalculable myriads of millenniums . . . All my previous selves have their voices, echoes, promptings in me . . . Oh, incalculable times again shall I be born."
Jack London
Born 1876—San Francisco, California

"Our birth is but a sleep and a forgetting;
The Soul that rises with us, our life's Star,
Hath had elsewhere its setting
And cometh from afar."
William Wordsworth
Born 1770—Cockermouth, UK

"Death is not the greatest loss in life. It's what dies inside while still alive."
Tupac Shakur
Born 1971—East Harlem, New York

"Oh, wow. Oh, wow. Oh, wow."
(final words)
Steve Jobs
Born 1955—San Francisco, California

"Grief, I've learned is really just love. It's all the love you want to give, but cannot. All that unspent love gathers up in the corners of your eyes, the lump of your throat, and in that hollow part of your chest. Grief is just love with no place to go."
Jamie Anderson
Born 1985—Reading, United Kingdom

XI

FAITH

"Always believe that something
wonderful is about to happen."
Coco Chanel
Born 1883—Saumur, France

"We all have our own life to pursue, our own kind of
dream to be weaving, and we all have the power to
make wishes come true, as long as we keep believing."
Louisa May Alcott
Born 1832—Philadelphia, Pennsylvania

"Faith is an oasis in the heart which will never
be reached by the caravan of thinking."
Khalil Gibran
Born 1883—Bsharri, Lebanon

"Faith is taking the first step, even when
you don't see the whole staircase."
Martin Luther King, Jr.
Born 1929—Atlanta, Georgia

"Faith is the bird that feels the light
when the dawn is still dark."
Rabindranath Tagore
Born 1861—Kolkata India

"Without faith a man can do nothing;
with it all things are possible."
Sir William Osler
Born 1849—Ontario, Canada

"Faith is the substance of things hoped for,
the evidence of things not seen."
Hebrews 11:1

"No coward soul is mine, no trembler in the world's
storm-troubled sphere; I see heaven's glories shine,
and faith shines equal, arming me from fear."
Emily Bronte
Born 1818—Haworth, United Kingdom

"What is faith unless it is to believe what you do not see?"
St. Augustine
Born 354—Thagaste, Algeria

"Faith is the strength by which a shattered
world shall emerge into the light."
Helen Keller
Born 1880—Tuscumbia, Alabama

XII

FORGIVENESS

"Forgiveness is the fragrance that the violet
sheds on the heel that has crushed it."
Mark Twain
Born 1835—Florida, Missouri

"Forgiveness is not always easy. At times, it
feels more painful than the wound we suffered,
to forgive the one that inflicted it. And yet,
there is no peace without forgiveness."
Marianne Williamson
Born 1952—Houston, Texas

"For every minute you remain angry, you give
up sixty seconds of peace of mind."
Ralph Waldo Emerson
Born 1803—Boston, Massachusetts

"Always forgive your enemies;
nothing annoys them so much."
Oscar Wilde
Born 1854—Dublin, Ireland

> "When another person makes you suffer,
> it is because he suffers deeply within himself,
> and his suffering is spilling over."
> **Thich Nhat Hanh**
> *Born 1926—Hue, Vietnam*

> "Ho' oponopono"
> *I'm sorry, forgive me, thank you. I love you.*
> **Ancient Hawaiian Forgiveness Prayer**

> "Haters are confused admirers who can't
> understand why everybody else likes you."
> **Paulo Coelho**
> *Born 1947—Rio de Janeiro, Brazil*

> "True forgiveness is when you can say
> thank you for that experience."
> **Oprah Winfrey**
> *Born 1954—Kosciusko, Mississippi*

> "There are only two ways to have a peaceful conscience:
> 1. Never do anything wrong 2. Learn self-forgiveness
> (pro tip: the first way's impossible)."
> **Eilzabeth Gilbert**
> *Born 1969—Waterbury, Connecticut*

> "To err is human; to forgive, divine."
> **Alexander Pope**
> *Born 1688—London, United Kingdom*

XIII

FRIENDSHIP

"Of all the things which wisdom provides to make us entirely happy, much the greatest is the possession of friendship."
Epicurus
Born 341 B.C.—Samos, Greece

"There is no wilderness like a life without friends; friendship multiplies blessings and minimizes misfortunes; it is a unique remedy against adversity, and it soothes the soul."
Baltasar Gracian
Born 1601—Belmonte de Gracian, Spain

"A good friend is the purest of all God's gifts."
Frances Farmer
Born 1913—Seattle, Washington

"Life is to be fortified by many friendships. To love, and to be loved, is the greatest happiness of existence."
Sydney Smith
Born 1771—London, United Kingdom

"A friend is someone who knows the song in your heart and can sing it back to you when you have forgotten the words."
Shania Twain
Born 1965—Windsor, Canada

"But friendship is precious, not only in the shade, but in the sunshine of life, and thanks to a benevolent arrangement the greater part of life is sunshine."
Thomas Jefferson
Born 1743—Shadwell, Virginia

"A friend is someone who understands your past, believes in your future, and accepts you today just the way you are."
Bernard Meltzer
Born 1916—New York, New York

"The growth of friendship is a lifelong affair."
Sarah Orne Jewett
Born 1849—South Berwick, Maine

"True happiness consists not in the multitude of friends, but in the worth and choice."
Ben Johnson
Born 1572—London, United Kingdom

XIV

GOD

"In music, in the sea, in a flower, in a leaf,
in an act of kindness . . . I see what
people call God in all these things."
Pablo Casals
Born 1876—Vendrell, Spain

"All major religious traditions carry basically the same
message, that is love, compassion and forgiveness. The
important thing is they should be part of our daily lives."
14th Dalai Lama
Born 1935—Taktser, China

"I cannot conceive how a man could look up
into the heavens and say there is no God."
Abraham Lincoln
Born 1809—Hodgenville, Kentucky

"I try to avoid looking forward or backward,
and try to keep looking upward."
Charlotte Bronte
Born 1816—Thornton, United Kingdom

> "My primary and most essential goal in life is to remain connected to the world of spirit. Everything else will take care of itself—this I know for sure."
> **Oprah Winfrey**
> *Born 1954—Kosciusko, Mississippi*

> "Allow your heart to expand and overflow with adoration for this magnificent creation and for the love, wisdom, and power that birthed it all."
> **Ann Mortifee**
> *Born 1947—Durban, South Africa*

> "Happiness keeps you sweet. Trials keep you strong. Sorrows keep you human. Failures keep you humble. Success keeps you growing. But only God keeps you going."
> **B.J. Morbitzer**
> *Born 1943—Columbus, Ohio*

> "The first peace, which is the most important, is that which comes within the souls of people when they realize their relationship, their oneness with the universe and all its powers, and when they realize at the center of the universe dwells the Great Spirit, and its center is really everywhere, it is within each of us."
> **Black Elk**
> *Born 1863—Powder River, Montana*

XV

GRATITUDE

"He is a wise man who does not grieve
for the things which he has not, but
rejoices for those which he has."
Epictetus
Born 50—Hierapolis, Turkey

"If the only prayer you say in your entire
life is *Thank You*, it will be enough."
Meister Eckhart
Born 1260—Gotha, Germany

"Appreciation is a wonderful thing. It makes what is
excellent in others belong to us as well."
Voltaire
Born 1694—Paris, France

"Today I consider myself the luckiest man on the face
of the Earth . . . I might have been given a bad
break, but I've got an awful lot to live for."
Lou Gehrig
Born 1903—New York, New York

> "One of the most tragic things I know about human nature is that all of us tend to put off living. We are all dreaming of some magical rose garden over the horizon—instead of enjoying the roses that are blooming outside our windows today."
>
> **Dale Carnegie**
> *Born 1888—Maryville, Missouri*

> Things turn out best for people who make the best of the way things turn out."
>
> **John Wooden**
> *Born 1910—Hall, Indiana*

> "The thankful heart opens our eyes to a multitude of blessings that continually surround us."
>
> **James E. Faust**
> *Born 1920—Delta, Utah*

> "Start each day with a grateful heart."
>
> **Psalm 107:1**

> "Barn's burnt down / Now I can see the moon."
>
> **Mizuta Masahide**
> *Born 1657—Zeze, Oomi*

XVI

HAPPINESS

"Happiness is the meaning and the purpose of life, the whole aim of human existence."
Aristotle
Born 384 B.C.—Stagira, Greece

"Happiness is pretty simple: someone to love, something to do, something to look forward to."
Rita Mae Brown
Born 1944—Hanover, Pennsylvania

"Happiness is a perfume you cannot pour on others without getting a few drops on yourself."
Ralph Waldo Emerson
Born 1803—Boston, Massachusetts

"Let us be grateful to the people who make us happy; they are the charming gardeners who make our souls blossom."
Marcel Proust
Born 1871—Paris, France

"The happiest person is the person who thinks the most interesting thoughts."
Timothy Dwight
Born 1828—Norwich, Connecticut

"Most folks are about as happy as they make up their minds to be."
Abraham Lincoln
Born 1809—Hodgenville, Kentucky

"Happiness not in another place, but this place, not for another hour, but this hour."
Walt Whitman
Born 1819—West Hills, New York

"Happiness resides not in possessions, and not in gold, happiness dwells in the soul."
Democritus
Born 460 B.C.—Abdera, Greece

"Happiness lies in the joy of achievement and the thrill of creative effort."
Franklin D. Roosevelt
Born 1882—Hyde Park, New York

"Humor is mankind's greatest blessing."
Mark Twain
Born 1835—Florida, Missouri

XVII

HOME/FAMILY

"He is happiest, be he a king or peasant,
who finds his peace in his home."
Johann Wolfgang von Goethe
Born 1749—Frankfurt, Germany

"A family is where character is formed, values are
learned, ethics are created, and society is preserved."
Manny Feldman
Born 1927—Newburgh, New York

"Family isn't always blood, it's the people in your life
who want you in theirs; the ones who accept you for
who you are, the ones who would do anything to see
you smile and who love you no matter what."
Maya Angelou
Born 1928—St. Louis, Missouri

"At the end only two things really matter to a man . . .
the affection and understanding of his family."
Richard E. Byrd
Born 1888—Winchester, Virginia

> "There's no place like home, there's no place like home, there's no place like home."
> **Frank Baum**
> *Born 1856—Chitennango, New York*

> "The more one does and sees and feels, the more one is able to do, and the more genuine may be one's appreciation of fundamental things like home, and love, and understanding companionship."
> **Amelia Earhart**
> *Born 1897—Atchison, Kansas*

> "To be a parent is to be a chief designer of a product more advanced than any technology and more interesting than any work of art."
> **Alain de Botton**
> *Born 1969—Zurich, Switzerland*

> "When you're safe at home you wish you were having an adventure; when you're having an adventure you wish you were safe at home."
> **Thorton Wilder**
> *Born 1897—Madison, Wisconsin*

> "Home is where the heart is."
> **Pliny**
> *Born 23—Cuomo, Italy*

XVIII

HOPE

"There was never a night or a problem
that could defeat sunrise or hope."
Bernard Williams
Born 1929—Westcliff-on-Sea, United Kingdom

"Never lose hope, my heart,
miracles dwell in the invisible."
Rumi
Born 1207—Balkh, Afghanistan

"The grand essentials to happiness in this life
are something to do, something to love,
and something to hope for."
Joseph Addison
Born 1672—Milston, United Kingdom

"It is necessary to hope . . . for hope itself is happiness."
Samuel Johnson
Born 1709—Lichfield, United Kingdom

> "Hold fast to dreams,
> For if dreams die
> Life is a broken-winged bird,
> That cannot fly."
>
> **Langston Hughes**
> *Born 1902—Joplin, Missouri*

> "Optimism is the faith that leads to achievement. Nothing can be done without hope and confidence."
>
> **Helen Keller**
> *Born 1880—Tuscumbia, Alabama*

> "Hope is never so lost it can't be found."
>
> **Ernest Hemingway**
> *Born 1899—Oak Park, Illinois*

> "Love recognizes no barriers. It jumps hurdles, leaps fences, penetrates walls to arrive at its destination full of hope."
>
> **Maya Angelou**
> *Born 1928—St. Louis, Missouri*

XIX

HUMBLENESS

"Talent is God given. Be humble.
Fame is man-given. Be grateful.
Conceit is self-given. Be careful."
John Wooden
Born 1910—Hall, Indiana

"Humility isn't thinking less of yourself,
but thinking of yourself less often."
C.S. Lewis
Born 1898—Belfast, Ireland

"The first product of self-knowledge is humility."
Flannery O'Connor
Born 1925—Savannah, Georgia

"Live so as to be detached from outcome. Do it all
because it resonates with your highest self—not
because of rewards that might come your way."
Wayne Dyer
Born 1940—Detroit, Michigan

"Hold the door, say please, say thank you.
Don't cheat, don't steal, and don't lie.
I know you got mountains to climb,
but always stay humble and kind."
Tim McGraw
Born 1967—Delhi, Louisiana

"Remembering that I'll be dead soon is the most important tool I've ever encountered to help me make the big choices in life. Because almost everything—all external expectations, all pride, all fear of embarrassment or failure—these things just fall away in the face of death, leaving only what is truly important."
Steve Jobs
Born 1955—San Francisco, California

"If you are humble nothing will touch you, neither praise, nor disgrace, because you know what you are."
Mother Teresa
Born 1910—Skopje, North Macedonia

XX

INTUITION

"Put your ear down close to your soul and listen hard."
Anne Sexton
Born 1928—Newton Massachusetts

"Your intuition always whispers. It very rarely shouts. If you can listen to the whisper, and if it tickles your heart, and is something you think you want to do for the rest of your life, then that is going to be what you do for the rest of your life, and we will benefit from everything you do."
Steven Spielberg
Born 1946—Cincinnati, Ohio

"Your heart knows the way, run in that direction."
Rumi
Born 1207—Balkh, Afghanistan

"Intuition is a very powerful thing, more powerful than intellect in my opinion."
Steve Jobs
Born 1955—San Francisco, California

"Your light. The one that goes blink, blink, inside your chest when you know what you're doing is right. Listen to it. Trust it. Let it make you stronger than you are."
Cheryl Strayed
Born 1968—Spangler, Pennsylvania

"Follow your instincts. That's where true wisdom manifests itself."
Oprah Winfrey
Born 1954—Kosciusko, Mississippi

"The intuitive mind is a sacred gift and the rational mind is a faithful servant. We have created a society that honors the servant and has forgotten the gift."
Albert Einstein
Born 1879—Ulm, Germany

"No teacher, preacher, parent, friend or wise man can decide what's right for you—just listen to the voice that speaks inside."
Shel Silverstein
Born 1930—Chicago, Illinois

"At the center of your being you have the answer; you know who you are and you know what you want."
Lao-Tzu
Born 571 B.C.—Chu, China

JOY

"A joyful heart is good medicine."
Proverbs 17:22

"Doing good to others is not a duty. It is a joy,
for it increases your own health and happiness."
Zoroaster
Born 628 B.C.—Airyanem Vaejah

"For me, life is about being positive and hopeful,
choosing to be joyful, choosing to be encouraging,
choosing to be empowering."
Billy Porter
Born 1969—Pittsburgh, Pennsylvania

"Find out where joy resides and give it a voice far
beyond singing. For to miss the joy is to miss all."
Robert Louis Stevenson
Born 1850—Edinburgh, United Kingdom

"In laughter, there is always a kind of joyousness
that is incompatible with contempt or indignation."
Voltaire
Born 1694—Paris, France

"The most important thing is to enjoy your
life—to be happy. It's all that matters."
Audrey Hepburn
Born 1929—Brussels, Belgium

"Think of the most wonderful experiences of your life:
your happiest moments, the supernatural episodes of
enhanced consciousness, the peak experiences when you
felt the highest levels of joy, harmony, and possibility."
Abraham Maslow
Born 1908—Brooklyn, New York

"Joy is a prayer, joy is strength, joy is love; joy
is a net of love by which you can catch souls."
Mother Teresa
Born 1910—Skopje, North Macedonia

"Find a place inside where there's joy,
and the joy will burn out the pain."
Joseph Campbell
Born 1904—White Plains, New York

XXII

KINDNESS

"No act of love however small, is ever wasted."
Aesop
Born 620 B.C.—Delphi, Greece

"I think probably kindness is my number one attribute in a human being. I'll put if before any of the things like courage or bravery or generosity or anything else. To be kind—it covers everything, to my mind. If you're kind that's it."
Roald Dahl
Born 1916—Cardiff, United Kingdom

"When given the choice between being right or being kind, always choose kind."
Wayne Dyer
Born 1940—Detroit, Michigan

"Do unto others as you would have them do unto you."
Luke 6:31

> "It is one of the most beautiful compensations of this life that no man can sincerely try to help another without helping himself."
> **Ralph Waldo Emerson**
> *Born 1803—Boston, Massachusetts*

> "There is no charm equal to tenderness of heart."
> **Jane Austen**
> *Born 1775—Steventon, United Kingdom*

> "Be kind whenever possible. It is always possible."
> **14th Dalai Lama**
> *Born 1935—Taktser, China*

> "We make a living by what we get. We make a life by what we give."
> **Sir Winston Churchill**
> *Born 1874—Blenheim, United Kingdom*

> "He that does good to another does also good to himself, not only in the consequence but in the very act. For the consciousness of well-doing is in itself ample reward."
> **Seneca**
> *Born 4 B.C.—Cordoba, Spain*

XXIII

LETTING GO

"Find the courage to let go of what you can't change."
Rumi
Born 1207—Balkh, Afghanistan

"You move on when your heart finally
understands there is no turning back."
J.R.R. Tolkien
Born 1892—Bloemfontein, South Africa

"If you're brave enough to say goodbye,
life will reward you with a new hello."
Paulo Coelho
Born 1947—Rio de Janeiro, Brazil

"To let go does not mean to get rid of. To let go
means to let be. When we let be with compassion
things come and go on their own."
Jack Kornfield
Born 1945—Philadelphia, Pennsylvania

"Life is like a river. If you cannot let go of the past, it will drag you down the stream."
Amit Ray
Born 1960—Calcutta, India

"In the process of letting go you will lose many things from the past, but you will find yourself."
Deepak Chopra
Born 1946—New Delhi, India

"Remember that not getting what you want is sometimes a wonderful stroke of luck."
14th Dalai Lama
Born 1935—Taktser, China

"Learning to let go of expectations is a ticket to peace."
Martha Beck
Born 1962—Provo, Utah

XXIV

LIFE PURPOSE

"Tell me, what is it you plan to do with
your one wild and precious life?"
Mary Oliver
Born 1935—Cleveland, Ohio

"I get up every morning determined to both change
the world and have one hell of a good time.
Sometimes this makes planning my day difficult."
E.B. White
Born 1899—Mount Vernon, New York

"Believe that maybe you too could add something
that would last and be beautiful."
Arthur Miller
Born 1915—Harlem, New York

"Dost thou love life?
Then do not squander time;
For that is the stuff life is made of."
Benjamin Franklin
Born 1706—Boston, Massachusetts

> "Those who have a 'why' to live,
> can bear with almost any 'how'."
> **Viktor E. Frankl**
> *Born 1905—Vienna, Austria*

> "Blessed is the man who has some congenial work, some occupation in which he can put his heart, and which affords a complete outlet to all the forces there are in him."
> **John Burroughs**
> *Born 1837—Roxbury, New York*

> "All that truly matters in this lifetime is the difference we make in the lives of others."
> **Cathy Byrd**
> *Born 1967—Pine Bluff, Arkansas*

> "Whatever you can do or dream you can, begin it. Boldness has genius, power, and magic in it."
> **Johann Wolfgang von Goethe**
> *Born 1749—Frankfurt, Germany*

> "Everybody has a creative potential and from the moment you can express this creative potential, you can start changing the world."
> **Paulo Coelho**
> *Born 1947—Rio de Janeiro, Brazil*

LIFE IS A MIRACLE

"When you are inspired by some great purpose, some extraordinary project, all your thoughts break their bonds: Your mind transcends limitations, your consciousness expands in every direction, and you find yourself in a new, great and wonderful world. Dormant forces, faculties and talents become alive, and you discover yourself to be a greater person by far than you ever dreamed yourself to be."
Patanjali
Born 200 B.C.—Kashmir, India

"Tame the savageness of man and make gentle the life of this world."
Aeschylus
Born 525—Eleusis, Greece

"Service makes our talents bear fruit and gives meaning to our lives. Those who do not live to serve, serve for little in this life."
Pope Francis
Born 1936—Buenos Aires, Argentina

"Whatever you decide to do, make sure it makes you happy."
Paulo Coelho
Born 1947—Rio de Janeiro, Brazil

XXV

LOVE

"The foundation of life is love and respect."
Tommy Lasorda
Born 1927—Norristown, Pennsylvania

"Love bears all things, believes all things, hopes all things, endures all things. Love never ends."
1 Corinthians 13: 7-8

"You yourself, as much as anybody in the entire universe, deserve your love and affection."
Buddha
Born 563 B.C.—Lumbini Province, Nepal

"Sometimes the smallest things take up the most room in your heart."
A.A. Milne
Born 1882—Hampstead, United Kingdom

"All that we love deeply becomes a part of us."
Helen Keller
Born 1880—Tuscumbia, Alabama

LIFE IS A MIRACLE

"Love is the bridge between you and everything."
Rumi
Born 1207—Balkh, Afghanistan

"Love is the greatest healing power I know. Love can heal even the deepest and most painful memories because love brings the light of understanding to the darkest corners of our hearts and minds."
Louise Hay
Born 1926—Los Angeles, California

"Life without love is like a tree without blossoms or fruit."
Kahlil Gibran
Born 1883—Bsharri, Lebanon

"I wish I'd known earlier in my life the importance of saying 'I love you.' You'd be surprised how many people don't really know how much they're loved."
Maria Shriver
Born 1955—Chicago, Illinois

"Tis better to have loved and lost, than never to have loved at all."
Alfred Lord Tennyson
Born 1809—Somersby, United Kingdom

XXVI

MANIFESTATION

"Every dream fulfilled begins with a simple wish."
Wayne Dyer
Born 1940—Detroit, Michigan

"The only thing that stands between a man and what he wants from life is often merely the will to try it and the faith to believe that it is possible."
Richard Devos
Born 1926—Grand Rapids, Michigan

"Stay strong and confident in your choices. Good things will come."
Monica Kirchner
Born 1971—Los Angeles, California

"When you want something, all the universe conspires in helping you to achieve it."
Paulo Coelho
Born 1947—Rio de Janeiro, Brazil

> "Build, therefore, your own world. As fast as you conform your life to the pure idea in your mind, that will unfold in its great proportions."

Ralph Waldo Emerson
Born 1803—Boston, Massachusetts

> "All our dreams can come true, if we have the courage to pursue them."

Walt Disney
Born 1901—Chicago, Illinois

> "Everything comes to us that belongs to us if we create the capacity to receive it."

Rabindranath Tagore
Born 1861—Kolkata India

> "You'll see it when you believe it."

Wayne Dyer
Born 1940—Detroit, Michigan

> "There is a law in psychology that if you form a picture in your mind of what you would like to be, and you keep and hold that picture long enough, you will soon become exactly as you have been thinking."

William James
Born 1842—New York, New York

XXVII

THE MIND

"The mind is its own place, and in itself can make a Heaven of hell, a hell of Heaven."
John Milton
Born 1608—London, United Kingdom

"As a man thinketh in his heart, so shall he be."
James Allen
Born 1864—Leicester, United Kingdom

"Very little is needed to make a happy life; it is all within yourself, in your way of thinking."
Marcus Aurelius
Born 121—Rome, Italy

"Heaven on Earth is a choice you must make, not a place you must find."
Wayne Dyer
Born 1940—Detroit, Michigan

LIFE IS A MIRACLE

"Have a mind that is open to everything,
and attached to nothing."
Tilopa
Born 988—Bengal, India

"Learning is an ornament in prosperity, a refuge
in adversity, and a provision in old age."
Aristotle
Born 384 B.C.—Stagira, Greece

"Things turn out best for people who make
the best of the way things turn out."
John Wooden
Born 1910—Hall, Indiana

"If you change the way you look at things,
the things you look at change."
Wayne Dyer
Born 1940—Detroit, Michigan

"Whether you think you can or
think you can't, you're right."
Henry Ford
Born 1863—Dearborn, Michigan

"Men are disturbed not by things that happen,
but by their opinions of the things that happen."
Epictetus
Born 55—Pamukkale, Turkey

"Pay no mind to the jealous ones."
Cathy Byrd
Born 1967—Pine Bluff, Arkansas

"To become the spectator of one's own life
is to escape the suffering of life."
Oscar Wilde
Born 1854—Dublin, Ireland

"Very little is needed to make a happy life.
It is all within yourself, in your way of thinking."
Marcus Aurelius
Born 121—Rome, Italy

XXVIII

MYSTERY OF LIFE

"Science cannot solve the ultimate mystery of nature. And that is because, in the last analysis, we ourselves are a part of the mystery that we are trying to solve."
Max Planck
Born 1858—Kiel, Germany

"Love is the answer, at least for most of the questions in my heart. Like why are we here? And where do we go? And how come it's so hard?"
Jack Johnson
Born 1975—North Shore, Hawaii

"Trust life, and it will teach you, in joy and sorrow, all you need to know."
James Baldwin
Born 1924—Harlem, New York

"Don't look for miracles. You are the miracle."
Henry Miller
Born 1891—Yorkville, New York

"The most beautiful thing we can experience is the mysterious. It is the source of all true art and science. He to whom this emotion is a stranger, who can no longer pause to wonder and stand rapt in awe, is as good as dead; his eyes are closed."
Albert Einstein
Born 1879—Ulm, Germany

"Every good and perfect gift is from above."
James 1:17

"I have observed the power of the watermelon seed. It has the power of drawing from the ground and through itself 200,000 times its weight. When you can explain to me the mystery of a watermelon, you can ask me to explain the mystery of God."
William Jennings Bryan
Born 1860—Salem, Illinois

XXIX

NATURE

"Study nature, love nature, stay close
to nature. It will never fail you."
Frank Lloyd Wright
Born 1867—Richland Center, Wisconsin

"Listen to the wind, it talks. Listen to the silence,
it speaks. Listen to your heart, it knows."
Native American Proverb

"Keep close to nature's heart . . . and break clear away,
once in a while, and climb a mountain or spend a
week in the woods. Wash your spirit clean."
John Muir
Born 1838—Dunbar, United Kingdom

"The answers to your problems lie all around you; in
each sunset, each pair of eyes, each breath of fresh air.
Find the beauty of nature and you have found your soul."
Vironika Tugaleva
Born 1988—Donetsk, Ukraine

"The butterfly counts not months but
moments, and has time enough."
Rabindranath Tagore
Born 1861—Kolkata India

"Even the darkest nights will end and the sun will rise."
Victor Hugo
Born 1802—Besancon, France

"The seeds you plant today will be the fruit you produce
in the future. What you plant will grow. Be mindful."
Trent Shelton
Born 1984—Little Rock, Arkansas

"Row, row, row your boat, gently down the stream,
merrily, merrily, merrily, merrily, life is but a dream."
Eliphalet Oram Lyte
Born 1842—Millersville, Pennsylvania

"If you expect the world to be fair with you because
you are fair, you are fooling yourself. That's like to expect
the lion not to eat you because you didn't eat him."
Paulo Coelho
Born 1947—Rio de Janeiro, Brazil

"The way I see it. If you want the rainbow
you gotta put up with the rain."
Dolly Parton
Born 1946—Locust Ridge, Tennessee

LIFE IS A MIRACLE

"The storm has the power to produce new
life, new beginnings, and new growth.
Find the purpose in the pain."
Trent Shelton
Born 1984—Little Rock, Arkansas

"Try to be like the turtle--at ease in your own shell."
Bill Copeland
Born 1946—Druid Hills, Georgia

"Clouds come floating into my life, no longer to carry
rain or usher storm, but to add color to my sunset sky."
Rabindranath Tagore
Born 1861—Kolkata India

"Nature does not hurry, yet everything is accomplished."
Lao-Tzu
Born 571 B.C.—Chu, China

"You cannot judge a tree or a person by only one season.
The essence of who they are, and the pleasure, joy, and
love that come from life, can only be measured at the end,
when all the seasons are up. If you give up when it's
winter, you will miss the promise of your spring, the
beauty of your summer and the fulfillment of your fall."
B.J Morbitzer
Born 1943—Columbus, Ohio

XXX

PEACE

"Peace will come to the hearts of men when they realize their oneness with the universe, it is everywhere."
Black Elk
Born 1863—Powder River, Montana

"And the peace of God which surpasses all understanding will guard your heart and mind."
Philippians 4:7

"Nothing can bring you peace but yourself."
Ralph Waldo Emerson
Born 1803—Boston, Massachusetts

"Undisturbed calmness of mind is attained by cultivating friendliness toward the happy, compassion for the unhappy, delight in the virtuous, and indifference toward the wicked."
Patanjali
Born 200 B.C.—Kashmir, India

"Music is the language of the spirit. It opens the secret of life bringing peace, abolishing strife."
Khalil Gibran
Born 1883—Bsharri, Lebanon

"What lies behind you and what lies in front of you pales in comparison to what lies inside of you."
Ralph Waldo Emerson
Born 1803—Boston, Massachusetts

"When a man achieves a fair measure of harmony within himself and his family circle, he achieves peace; and a nation made up of such individuals and groups is a happy nation."
Richard E. Byrd
Born 1888—Winchester, Virginia

"Money may be the husk of many things, but not the kernel.
It brings you food, but not appetite; medicine, but not health; acquaintances, but not friends; servants, but not faithfulness; days of joy, but not peace or happiness."
Henrik Ibsen
Born 1828—Skien, Norway

XXXI

PERSEVERANCE

"With everything that has happened to you, you can either feel sorry for yourself, or treat what has happened as a gift. Everything is either an opportunity to grow or an obstacle to keep you from growing. You get to choose."
Wayne Dyer
Born 1940—Detroit, Michigan

"The difference between the impossible and the possible lies in a person's determination."
Tommy Lasorda
Born 1927—Norristown, Pennsylvania

"Fall seven times and stand up eight."
Japanese Proverb

"A great pleasure in life is to do what they say you can't."
Paulo Coelho
Born 1947—Rio de Janeiro, Brazil

LIFE IS A MIRACLE

"The most difficult thing is the decision to
act, the rest is merely tenacity."
Amelia Earhart
Born 1897—Atchison, Kansas

"If your problems feel big, climb to a mountaintop
and take another look. Perspective is everything."
Cathy Byrd
Born 1967—Pine Bluff, Arkansas

"I have been impressed with the urgency of doing.
Knowing is not enough; we must apply.
Being willing is not enough; we must do."
Leonardo da Vinci
Born 1452—Anchiano Italy

"Great works are performed not by
strength, but by perseverance."
Samuel Johnson
Born 1709—Lichfield, United Kingdom

"In the realm of ideas, everything depends on
enthusiasm; in the real world, all rests on perseverance."
Johann Wolfgang von Goethe
Born 1749—Frankfurt, Germany

"Mediocrity sucks."
Dr. Michael Becker
Born 1953—Kaiserslautern, Germany

"And this too shall pass."
Attar of Nishapur
Born 1146—Kadkan, Iran

"Be ready to pay the price of your dreams. Free cheese can only be found in a mouse trap."
Paulo Coelho
Born 1947—Rio de Janeiro, Brazil

"I've come to learn pain teaches more than hurt. The sun rise and rise and rise, it will rise again."
Stephen Marley
Born 1972—Wilmington, Delaware

XXXII

POSSIBILITY

"For you see, so many out-of-the-way things had happened lately, that Alice had begun to think that very few things indeed were really impossible."
Lewis Carroll
Born 1832—Daresbury, United Kingdom

"For with God nothing shall be impossible."
Luke 1:37

"The future belongs to those who believe in the beauty of their dreams."
Eleanor Roosevelt
Born 1884—New York, New York

"Risk more than others think is safe.
Care more than others think is wise.
Dream more than others think is practical.
Expect more than others think is possible."
Claude Bissell
Born 1916—Meaford, Ontario

> "Ask, and it shall be given you; seek, and ye shall find; knock, and it shall be opened unto you."
> **Matthew 7:7**

> "Nothing has ever been achieved by the person who says, 'It can't be done.'"
> **Eleanor Roosevelt**
> *Born 1884—New York, New York*

> "Today was good. Today was fun. Tomorrow is another one."
> **Dr. Seuss**
> *Born 1904—Springfield, Massachusetts*

> "It's the possibility of having a dream come true that makes life interesting."
> **Paulo Coelho**
> *Born 1947—Rio de Janeiro, Brazil*

> "Whatever the mind of man can conceive and believe, it can achieve."
> **Napoleon Hill**
> *Born 1883—Pound, Virginia*

> "You are not your circumstances.
> You are your possibilities.
> If you know that, you can do anything."
> **Oprah Winfrey**
> *Born 1954—Kosciusko, Mississippi*

XXXIII

PRAYERS

"This is my wish for you: Comfort on difficult days, smiles when sadness intrudes, rainbows to follow the clouds, laughter to kiss your lips, sunsets to warm your heart, hugs when spirits sag, beauty for your eyes to see, friendships to brighten your being, faith so that you can believe, confidence for when in doubt, courage to know yourself, patience to accept the truth, Love to complete your life."
Ralph Waldo Emerson
Born 1803—Boston, Massachusetts

"May the road rise to meet you.
May the wind be always be at your back.
May the sun shine warm upon your face,
and rains fall soft upon your fields.
And, until we meet again,
May God hold you in the palm of His hand."
The Irish Blessing
Author Unknown

"To believe is to know that
every day is a new beginning.
It is to trust that miracles happen,
and dreams really do come true.

To believe is to know the value of
a nurturing heart, the innocence
of a child's eyes and the beauty
of an aging hand, for it is through
their teachings, we learn how to love.

To believe is to find the strength
and courage that lies within us
when it's time to pick up the
pieces and begin again.

To believe is to know we are not
alone, that life is a gift and this is
our time to cherish it.

To believe is to know that
wonderful surprises are just
waiting to happen, and all our
hopes and dreams are within reach.
If only we believe."

B.J. Morbitzer
Born 1943—Columbus, Ohio

Peace Prayer of Saint Francis

"Lord, make me an instrument of your peace:
Where there is hatred,
Let me sow love;
Where there is injury, pardon;
Where there is doubt, faith;
Where there is despair, hope;
Where there is darkness, light;
And where there is sadness, joy.

O divine Master,
Grant that I may not so much seek
To be consoled as to console,
To be understood as to understand,
To be loved as to love.
For it is in giving that we receive,
It is in pardoning that we are pardoned,
And it is in dying
That we are born to eternal life."

St. Francis of Assisi
Born 1182—Assisi, Italy

Promise Yourself

"Promise yourself to be so strong that nothing can disturb your peace of mind. To talk health, happiness, and prosperity to every person you meet. To make all your friends feel that there is something in them. To look at the sunny side of everything and make your optimism come true. To think only the best, to work only for the best, and to expect only the best. To be just as enthusiastic about the success of others as you are about your own. To forget the mistakes of the past and press on to the greater achievements of the future. To wear a cheerful countenance at all times and give every living creature you meet a smile. To give so much time to the improvement of yourself that you have no time to criticize others. To be too large for worry, too noble for anger, too strong for fear, and too happy to permit the presence of trouble. To think well of yourself and to proclaim this fact to the world, not in loud words but great deeds. To live in faith that the whole world is on your side so long as you are true to the best that is in you."

Christian D. Larson
Born 1874—Forrest City, Iowa

XXXIV

SLEEP/DREAMS

"We often dream about people from whom we receive a letter by the next post. I have ascertained on several occasions that at the moment when the dream occurred the letter was already lying in the post-office of the addressee."
Carl Jung
Born 1875—Kesswil, Switzerland

"When we are asleep in this world, we are awake in another."
Salvador Dali
Born 1904—Figueres, Spain

"In a dream, in a vision of the night, when deep sleep falls upon men, while slumbering in their beds, then He opens the ears of men, and seals their instruction."
Job 33:15-16

"All that we see or seem, is but a dream within a dream."
Edgar Allan Poe
Born 1809—Boston, Massachusetts

> "The soul is silent.
> If it speaks at all
> It speaks in dreams."
> **Louise Gluck**
> *Born 1943—New York, New York*

> "Sleep is the time when your conscious mind leaves the world of your five senses and joins in with your subconscious mind. You spend one-third of your life sleeping and this is where you receive instructions for how the other two-thirds of your life can unfold. Here is where you receive the instructions for running your life smoothly, effortlessly, and miraculously."
> **Wayne Dyer**
> *Born 1940—Detroit, Michigan*

> "Trust the dreams, for in them
> is hidden the gate to eternity."
> **Kahlil Gibran**
> *Born 1883—Bsharri, Lebanon*

XXXV

SOLITUDE

"All man's troubles derive from not
being able to sit quietly in a room alone."
Blaise Pascal
Born 1623—Clermont-Ferrand, France

"God's one and only voice is silence."
Herman Melville
Born 1819—New York, New York

"Out beyond ideas of wrongdoing
and rightdoing there is a field.
I'll meet you there."
Rumi
Born 1207—Balkh, Afghanistan

"It takes solitude, under the stars,
for us to be reminded of our eternal
origin and our far destiny."
Archibald Rutledge
Born 1883—McClellanville, South Carolina

"The best thinking has been done in solitude."
Thomas A. Edison
Born 1847—Milan, Ohio

"Sometimes, the most profound of awakenings come wrapped in the quietest of moments."
Stephen Crane
Born 1871—Newark, New Jersey

"Silence and solitude, the soul's best friends."
Henry Wadsworth Longfellow
Born 1807—Portland, Maine

"The more you go within, the more you understand your true nature, and the more joy and happiness you feel in your life."
Brian Weiss
Born 1944—New York, New York

"Quiet the mind and the soul will speak."
Buddha
Born 563 B.C.—Lumbini Province, Nepal

XXXVI

SUCCESS

"To laugh often and much; to win the respect of intelligent people and the affection of children; to earn the appreciation of honest critics and to endure the betrayal of false friends. To appreciate beauty; to find the best in others; to leave the world a bit better whether by a healthy child, a garden patch, or a redeemed social condition; to know that even one life has breathed easier because you have lived. This is to have succeeded."
Ralph Waldo Emerson
Born 1803—Boston, Massachusetts

"Success is peace of mind which is a direct result of self-satisfaction in knowing you did your best to become the best you are capable of becoming."
John Wooden
Born 1910—Hall, Indiana

"Strive not to be a success, but rather to be of value."
Albert Einstein
Born 1879—Ulm, Germany

"Like success, failure is many things to many people. With positive mental attitude, failure is a learning experience, a rung on the ladder, a plateau at which to get your thoughts in order and prepare to try again."
Clement Stone
Born 1902—Chicago, Illinois

"No one has learned the meaning of living until he has surrendered his ego to the service of his fellow man."
Beran Wolfe
Born 1900—Vienna, Austria

"For our own success to be real, it must contribute to the success of others."
Eleanor Roosevelt
Born 1884—New York, New York

"Success is walking from failure to failure with no loss of enthusiasm."
Sir Winston Churchill
Born 1874—Blenheim, United Kingdom

"If one advances confidently in the direction of his dreams, and endeavors to live the life he has imagined, he will meet with a success unexpected in common hours."
Henry David Thoreau
Born 1817—Concord, Massachusetts

LIFE IS A MIRACLE

"Grow where you are planted
and success will find you."
Cathy Byrd
Born 1967—Pine Bluff, Arkansas

"You'll never see a U-Haul behind a hearse. Now,
I've been blessed to make hundreds of millions
of dollars in my life. I can't take it with me, and
neither can you. It's not how much you have,
but what you do with what you have."
Denzel Washington
Born 1954—Mount Vernon, New York

XXXVII

SYNCHRONICITY/MAGIC

"Pay attention to synchronicities and people who touch your life every day. These people can be angels who will help you along the way."
Dr. Wayne Dyer
Born 1940—Detroit, Michigan

"There are only two ways to live your life. One is as though nothing is a miracle. The other is as though everything is a miracle."
Albert Einstein
Born 1879—Ulm, Germany

"And above all, watch with glittering eyes the whole world around you because the greatest secrets are always hidden in the most unlikely places. Those who don't believe in magic will never find it."
Roald Dahl
Born 1916—Cardiff, UK

> "Synchronicity is the coming together of inner and outer events in a way that cannot be explained by cause and effect and that is meaningful to the observer."
>
> **Carl Jung**
> *Born 1875—Kesswil, Switzerland*

> "The world is full of magic things, patiently waiting for our senses to grow sharper."
>
> **W.B. Yeats**
> *Born 1865—Sandymount, Ireland*

> "Our brightest blazes of gladness are commonly kindled by unexpected sparks."
>
> **Samuel Johnson**
> *Born 1709—Lichfield, United Kingdom*

> "Our time here is magic! It's the only space you have to realize whatever it is that is beautiful, whatever is true, whatever is great, whatever is potential, whatever is rare, whatever is unique, in. It's the only space."
>
> **Ben Okri**
> *Born 1959—Minna, Nigeria*

> "Not all things in life need to be understood in order to be appreciated."
>
> **Cathy Byrd**
> *Born 1967—Pine Bluff, Arkansas*

"Don't give up before the miracle happens."
Fannie Flagg
Born 1944—Birmingham, Alabama

"If you could only sense how important you are to the lives of those you meet; how important you can be to the people you may never even dream of. There is something of yourself that you leave at every meeting with another person."
Fred Rogers
Born 1928—Latrobe, Pennsylvania

"There is a secret garden where miracles and magic abound, and it is available to anyone who makes the choice to visit there."
Dr. Wayne Dyer
Born 1940—Detroit, Michigan

"Your life will always be filled with delightful mysteries. Keep going and you will find them."
Cathy Byrd
Born 1967—Pine Bluff, Arkansas

EXTRAS

SALTWATER

"Everyone who terrifies you is sixty-five percent water.
And everyone you love is made of stardust,
and I know
sometimes
you cannot even breathe deeply, and
the night sky is no home, and
you have cried yourself to sleep enough times
that you are down to your last two percent, but
nothing is infinite,
not even loss.
You are made of the sea and the stars, and one day
you are going to find yourself again."

Finn Butler
Born 1995—London, United Kingdom
from her collection of poems, *From the Wreckage*

Do It Anyway

"People are often unreasonable, illogical and self-centered; *Forgive them anyway.*
If you are kind, people may accuse you of selfish, ulterior motives; *Be kind anyway.*
If you are successful, you will win some false friends and some true enemies; *Succeed anyway.*
If you are honest and frank, people may cheat you; *Be honest and frank anyway.*
What you spend years building, someone could destroy overnight; *Build anyway.*
If you find serenity and happiness, they may be jealous; *Be happy anyway.*
The good you do today, people will often forget tomorrow; *Do good anyway.*
Give the world the best you have, and it may never be enough; *Give the world the best you've got anyway.*
You see, in the final analysis, it is between you and your God; *It was never between you and them anyway.*"

Kent M. Keith
Born 1949—Brooklyn, New York

"A few things on my heart these days that I need say to you before the sun sets . . .

1. The people who come to steal your wonder are the same folks who long ago let others freely take theirs. Never let it go. It's yours. Cling to your sweetness and become a living witness to the million beautiful curiosities of your life. Don't let anything become mundane. Pay close attention to the adventure before you. All of your experiences are soaked in magic; the good and the bad, the happy and the sad, the hilarious and the mad.

2. Every time you see a mother holding her baby I want you to fall down the rabbit hole of creation's divine mastery. Babies are the key to the mystery of our entire experience here on earth. Don't let a baby pass by you without becoming bewildered by the whole wonderful oddity of life.

3. When your heart gets broken—and it will—I am begging you to count each tear that rolls down your face as the blessing that it is. You are crying because you haven't let your heart go numb. You are crying because you let yourself be vulnerable. You are crying because you are still fighting to stay alive. You are crying because you have accepted your humanity. Every tear is proof of how incredibly strong you are. Be proud of your shedding tears! Each tear is unique and telling your story drop by beautiful drop.

4. On the occasion when you find yourself watching a sunset please spend a fat second breathing in the last seconds of the dying light. Take a moment to learn the great lesson of twilight despite the long night. The light always returns and darkness always loses. The game is rigged.

5. Every breath you take is proof that your existence is a singular event. There will never be anybody else like you again. Everything you do makes history and every time you exhale it sends a fresh ripple through the galaxy. Listen, there is only one you. Every second that washes over you is something brand new that this universe has never seen before. Be fearless.

6. During the times when your stomach hurts from laughing so much with a friend, don't let the moment slip past without first acknowledging the unappreciated miracle of the soul friends you meet here on Earth. They are the same ones that you knew before you came into being. You knew each other before birth and promised to find one another down here in the blood and mud. Good work you two!

7. Someday we will hold hands for the last time, but if you let that moment take root inside of you it will last a thousand lifetimes. Let our fleeting time together grow into a towering redwood tree. Time is relentless, but it is no match for love. Honor every second of the clock; treat every little bit of your experience like the wild phenomenon that it is. Be a vigilant witness to the magic of everything.

8. Don't become forgetful of your dignity or that on the day you were born you were covered in the dust of first-day creation. You were forged out of the most brilliant of celestial fires. Never take for granted all of that radiates in you. You were born to blaze. Don't forget, don't forget, don't forget."

John Roedel
Born 1966—London, United Kingdom

> LIVE THE LIFE YOU'VE ALWAYS DREAMED OF. BE FEARLESS IN THE FACE OF ADVERSITY. NEVER STOP LEARNING. USE YOUR IMAGINATION WHENEVER POSSIBLE. RECOGNIZE THE **BEAUTY** THAT SURROUNDS **YOU**. REMEMBER WHERE YOU CAME FROM, BUT NEVER LOSE SIGHT OF WHERE YOU ARE GOING.

www.ingramcontent.com/pod-product-compliance
Lightning Source LLC
Chambersburg PA
CBHW072014290426
44109CB00018B/2240